Prayers beyond the CHEMO CHAIR

PRAISE, ENCOURAGEMENT & A TESTIMONY OF HEALING

SANDRA G. JONES

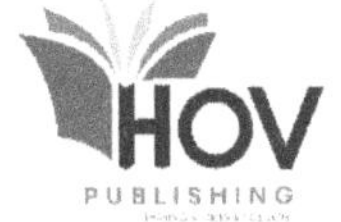

PRAYERS BEYOND THE CHEMO CHAIR

HOV Publishing a division of HOV, LLC.
www.hovpub.com
hopeofvision@gmail.com

Cover Design: Chantelle Roberts for Xcelled Designs
Editor: Amy Owens for Clarity Communications
Editor/Proofread: B. Walker Consulting

Contact the Author, Sandra G. Jones at:
sandrabennett903@gmail.com

For further information regarding special discounts on bulk purchases, please reply to www.hovpub.com

ISBN Paperback: 978-1-942871-81-1
ISBN eBook: 978-1-942871-82-8

10 9 8 7 6 5 4 3 2 1

Printed in the United States of America

Dedication

This book is dedicated to Rodney Wilkerson, Mary Slaughter, and Toni Bennett.

Prayers beyond the CHEMO CHAIR

Contents

1 Introduction

5 Prayers of Praise

27 Prayers of Glory

38 My Life Will Never Be the Same

41 My Days of Loneliness

42 Words of Encouragement

44 My Testimony

46 Let Me Preach

51 All the Glory Belongs to God!

53 About the Author

55 Praises, Encouragement, & Testimony Journal

Prayers beyond the
CHEMO CHAIR

Introduction

Born Sandra Gaston, Pastor Sandra G. Jones was diagnosed with Stage 2 Breast Cancer in 2011. When she first heard her doctor confirm the diagnosis, she was in shock but then began to pray. She quietly excused herself from the doctor's office (leaving her sister behind) and went into the restroom to privately consult with the Lord. The Lord revealed that this was a test of her faith—a test of faith that she would have to endure for the sake of her own spiritual growth and testimony to others.

"When you challenged like I was, you have to stay positive at all times," Pastor Jones said, "After all, you cannot trust God and doubt Him at the same time. Try meditating daily. Do not lie in bed all the time. Instead, get up and praise God for everything you see. Always remember, your life and destiny is already written, for God is the author and finisher of your faith."

My first day in the chemo chair left me feeling lonely and sad, even though I was not alone. My sister and aunt were there supporting me. I remember silently trying to console myself:

"God is with you and He will get you through this," I kept telling myself.

Satan set out to test my faith, but my love for God and the word of God would not allow me to give up. I kept reciting, *"thy faith hath made thee whole."* (Mark 5:34). I would much rather lose my mind than to lose my faith in God. And that nearly happened too but the Lord never left my side.

I advise anyone undergoing treatment for cancer to take things step-by-step. Know that God is right there with you. Stay in a close relationship with Christ, for He is your friend, brother, Lord, King, and most of all, a healer with all power in His hands. He is able to raise the dead, so fear nothing. Trust God and talk to Him throughout the process.

I thank God every day for my life and continue to do so to this very day. Believing in God's miracles made my faith stronger. I constantly read the Bible to remind myself of God's grace. I stay in prayer to remain covered and I learned to bless and give to others, so my Heavenly Father can bless me.

The nurses and doctors were on the job. I was on the job for the Lord. And God was on the job for my soul.

Surviving cancer is a fight. A fight that requires the right weapons:

- Love
- Faith
- Trust
- Patience
- Hope
- Peace
- Forgiveness

Make sure your heart is clean so your body can heal. Stay before the Lord in prayer. Know when to engage in battle and when to come out. You are not always on the front line and you are never alone. *"The Lord will fight for you, you need only to be still."* (Exodus 14:14, NIV).

Trust in the Lord when you are tired. He will give you the strength to stand. I pray that the prayers I prayed will be a blessing to your soul. God touched my soul and led me to share them with anyonc who is fighting the good fight of faith.

Again, I say, trust in the Lord. He will see you beyond the chemo chair. Know that I am praying for you. Although I only know you in spirit, I pray that you always remember that God is able!

Prayers beyond the CHEMO CHAIR

Prayers of Praise

Prayer of Praise #1

When I think of my Father and the God I serve, it reminds me of love. You, God, are many things: You are joy, happiness, peace, and most of all, love. From this great love comes blessings, grace, and mercy. Thank you, Lord for loving me unconditionally.

PRAISE HIM!

Always know that you are loved.

Prayer of Praise #2

Lord, forgive me for all my sins. May Your mercy shine upon my family and me. Only you, Lord Jesus, can know how hard the road is to walk. How far the way seems to be for me. I know not to give up because you are waiting on me with open arms. When Your people fall, they must get back up.

PRAISE HIM!

On the road of righteousness there awaits a fight. Satan is waiting for me to get tired. He wants me to give up. Thank you, God, for helping me stand and for allowing things to happen to get my attention. Hold my hands when I fall. Pull me out of the miry clay.

Prayer of Praise #3

Lord Jesus have mercy on me. My heart is hurt, and my spirit is low. Bring me into a place of peace and happiness. Help me to think more about my blessings, so I can praise you. Keep my mind off the things I cannot fix. Help me to know that You, Almighty God, have the power to do all things. You will take my bad and make it work for Your good. I will serve the Lord, who is able to change the path of my life and bless me with joy when faith seems impossible.

PRAISE HIM!

"Have mercy upon me, O Lord: for I am weak; Oh Lord heal me: for my bones are vexed." (Psalm 6:2)

Prayer of Praise #4

God will save me. He will lift me up out of sadness and stand me on my feet. I will walk with the joy and love of God. He has made it known that my tears are precious to him. "Cry no more, precious child," God says, "I will give you peace." Know that God is with you and that He is all powerful.

PRAISE HIM!

"Hear the voice of my supplications, when I cry unto thee..." (Psalm 28:2a)

Prayer of Praise #5

Lord, I have given love, yet I have kept a little for myself. My heart is big, but my sadness is long. Help me, Lord Jesus, to understand why the ones You love the most seem to hurt You the most.

The pain in my cup is running over. I am trying not to hate. I pray on my knees that God will help me to trust and love again. You have always been by my side. You read my heart. I am as real as I can be. Father, I hold You to Your promise that You will never leave me.

PRAISE HIM!

When I was on my sick bed and at the bottom of despair, I found comfort in You, Lord Jesus. *"Looking unto Jesus the author and finisher of our faith, who for the joy that was set before Him endured the cross."* (Hebrews 12:2).

Prayer of Praise #6

The Lord was in my spirit today. Thank you, almighty God for your Holy Spirit.

PRAISE HIM!

My help is not far. This I know. You, God will fight my battle for me, and victory will be mine. Isn't it funny how God can change things to work out for our good? We go through all types of things in order to line up with His will.

Prayer of Praise #7

All days will not be good, but if you trust God, they will get better. There is always sadness in our lives. We never know how we will feel from one day to another. One day we may be happy and the next day sad. Jesus doesn't want it that way. He wants us to have enough love in our hearts to be happy every day. Enough love to trust Him and know that it's going to be okay.

PRAISE HIM!

Prayer of Praise #8

Lord, when I woke up this morning, Satan tried to make me feel as if all types of illnesses were upon me. God, I know whatever You have for me it must be big—so big that Satan cannot tear it down. The Lord has healed me. I am blessed to receive such a big grace! I know this in my spirit!!!

PRAISE HIM!

Prayer of Praise #9

Lord, I thank you! Every day is getting better and better now that I've learned to let God fight my battles!

PRAISE HIM!

Be still! God will fight your battle. It is true.
Praise God!

Prayer of Praise #10

Lord, as I raise my head off my pillow this morning, I rise up with praise. I know that I have to praise my way through this day! Today, everything is coming at me at one time. God is with me as I cry out to Him. He already knows all things pertaining to my life.

The Savior I serve will fight my battles for me. In the same way my enemy took from me, God will restore all things to me. Though others may speak death, God will give me life.

If you cannot speak blessings and love, then speak nothing at all. Your words should come out of God's love. The love from my heart is real, and the God I serve is real too. He will reward me for the love and work I have done. He will also let me see the enemy fall and stand before me asking for forgiveness.

GIVE GOD THE PRAISE!

"I will cry unto God most high; unto God that performs all things for me." (Psalm 57:2)

Prayer of Praise #11

Lord, thank you Father, for hearing my prayer. You are always on time. I need a blessing so bad, and my soul cries out to You. My mouth does not have to be open for You to hear me. The God I serve will always be fair to His people.

PRAISE HIM!

Even when your mouth is unable to speak, He hears your heart.

Prayer of Praise #12

Oh Lord, what can I say to thee? You know everything about me. All my thoughts are with thee. When my heart is broken, you already know.

What can I hide from you? Nothing! My cup is half full. Fill me, Lord. My days are lonely. Please bring me the love of my wants and needs, so I may be happy and at peace with myself.

PRAISE HIM!

It's okay to cry out to the Lord.

Prayer of Praise #13

Lord, on my bad days, I call upon God to help me continue my fight. When I meditate on you, Father, and all that You have done for me I realize I am blessed to be able to stand in your presence. My help comes from You. Thank you God for loving me.

PRAISE HIM

Oh bless, His holy name!

Prayer of Praise #14

Praise God almighty! I thank you Lord, for loving me. Love is the greatest blessing that anyone can received. In order, for me to love like Jesus, the love of God has to first be in me. Thank you, oh God, for being a such a giving and forgiving God.

PRAISE HIM!

Even when we are feeling empty, He is still giving! Trust Him to get you through.

Prayer of Praise #15

Lord, my heart is tired, and my eyes are sleepy, but you, oh Lord, kept me awake to make it safely home. I have praised You for two hours. I have preached His word. Jesus has a way of reviving me. I feel refreshed.

PRAISE HIM!

God gave me the strength to preach His word.

Prayer of Praise #16

Heavenly Father, at times I wonder why people lie when the truth is so much easier to speak. Please forgive me if I have told a lie because the truth is freeing.

PRAISE HIM!

I love you, Jesus! People will lie to you while you are on your sick bed, but I pray for them that their hearts will change.

Prayer of Praise #17

Don't pay a price that is too high for you. Don't make a deal that becomes a bill. Let God guide you.

PRAISE HIM!

Remember, even when you are feeling better, Satan has a trick. Ask God to lead you.

Prayer of Praise #18

Lord, oh how I need thee to come and see about me. I need thee to brighten my spirit. I have been deceived long enough. They say that they are not liars but God knows the truth. Fight my battles for me. Let all the firing arrows that they shoot return to them with quickness. Let my love and your love be a shield for me. Let me behold God with my eyes daily.

PRAISE GOD ALMIGHTY!

This is the time to give praise. I will sing a song to the Lord.

Prayer of Praise #19

Oh, bless the Lamb of God. He is a keeper of His people. I called on your name and every round became easier. I can smile just thinking about your mercy.

PRAISE HIM!

"And He said unto her, Daughter, thy faith hath made thee whole; go in peace and be whole of thy plague." (Mark 5:34)

Prayer of Praise #20

God, this has not been easy but I made it through chemo, by trusting in You and holding onto Your healing hands. I know You will restore all that I have lost. God is a healer! He never left me!

PRAISE HIM!

"But when Jesus heard it, He answered him saying, fear not: believe only and she shall be made whole." (Luke 8:50)

Prayer of Praise #21

My fight with breast cancer has changed me in a way that caused me to have a closer and deeper relationship with God. I am closer to God now and I am moving into a deeper level of trust and faith in Him. As a Pastor, who almost lost her church, home, and bank account, I am closer to God now than ever before. My faith is stronger. I am a new creature in Christ. Sometimes we have to be stripped down to nothing to become what God has ordained us to be.

PRAISE HIM!

Because I chose life, I am holding onto God's unchanging hands. May God be your strength also. Put all your trust in God and stay positive. Remember, God is a healer of His people.

Prayers of Glory

Prayer of Glory #1

Lord God, my Father, thank You for staying by my side. Thank You for still moving upon this earth. I seek You and You are found. I knock and the door was opened. Now, help me to walk in my purpose. I will meet You at the water (the ocean) during a well needed trip.

GIVE GOD THE GLORY

"In the beginning God created the heavens and the earth. And the earth was without form, and void; and darkness was upon the face of the deep and the spirit of God moved upon the face of the waters." (Genesis 1:1-2)

Prayer of Glory #2

As I begin the new life, let me be untouchable by the enemy. When the enemy attacks my flesh, do not allow him to have any power over my body, life, or ministry. You alone are all powerful and all power lies in your hands.

GIVE GOD ALL THE GLORY

"No evil shall be allowed to befall you, no plague come near your tent." (Psalm 91:10)

Prayer of Glory #3

As I sit here thinking of the goodness of God, words can express my tears of joy. Only God, my Father, knows how thankful I am to be alive and present in His sight.

TO GOD BE ALL THE GLORY

"The thief cometh not, but for to steal, and to kill, and to destroy. I am come that they might have life, and that they might have it more abundantly." (John 10:10)

Prayer of Glory #4

Heavenly Father, I have been through the storm, been almost broken down to nothing, and left in a dry land. But you never left me alone. When I couldn't eat natural food, you fed me spiritual food. When I was unable to sleep, you talked to me all night. I knew in my heart that all was well by faith. Your Holy Spirit brought me through all my afflictions.

GIVE GOD THE GLORY

"Many are the afflictions of the righteous, but the Lord delivers him out of them all." (Psalm 34:19)

Prayer of Glory #5

What an awesome God we serve! Father, as I humble myself before You—the Most High God—I am safe, I am loved, and I am covered under Your blood. Lord, I thank You. My journey was filled with light and I am winning this fight. Bless the Lamb of God.

GIVE GOD THE GLORY

"How excellent is thy loving kindness, O God therefore, the children of men put their trust under the shadow of thy wings." (Psalm 36:7)

Prayer of Glory #6

Allow me to thank You, Lord God, for being real in my life. I have never questioned the work of God because my faith would seem weak. I knew the Lord would get me through all this. Praise your name, Jesus. Bless the Lamb of God.

GIVE GOD THE GLORY

"And Jesus looking upon them saith, with man it is impossible, but not with God; for with God all things are possible." (Matthew 19:26)

Prayer of Glory #7

My praise and worship are not good enough, for all the blessings He has given me. But it is my desire to stay in the presence of God. I have a friend like no other. His name is Jesus and He has been by my side all the way. Oh, how I love Him.

GIVE GOD THE GLORY

"But the hour cometh and now is when the true worshippers shall worship the Father in spirit and in truth: for the Father seeketh such to worship Him." (John 4:23)

Prayer of Glory #8

God has a way of building up our strength. Lord, I know sometimes You have to take us to the bottom to get us to the top. For that, Lord, I thank You.

GIVE GOD THE GLORY

"Jesus saith unto him rise, take up thy bed and walk." (John 5:8)

Prayer of Glory #9

Lord God, You are Holy. You are Powerful. You are Almighty. I praise You, God, for covering me in the blood of Jesus. When I thought I could not make it, Your love said, "I got this!" When I could not eat your word, You fed me. When I could not sleep, You gave me rest. Oh, how sweet it is to be kept by Jesus.

GIVE GOD THE GLORY

"Giving thanks always for all things unto God and the Father in the name of our Lord, Jesus Christ." (Ephesians 5:20)

Testimony of Healing

My Life Will Never Be The Same

As I stepped into the chemo room not knowing what to expect, I began to talk to Jesus in my spirit. Lord, I never thought so many people could fit in one room. "Lord why is cancer attacking so many people?" I asked in silence, as I took in the atmosphere before me.

I could only take two family members into the chemo room with me. The nurse asked me to pick a chair. The treatments were four hours each day. There were 25 chemo recliners. Everyone was lined up. Some people were sitting and reading. Some were talking as if they looked forward to seeing each other. Still, others were sitting alone crying. "My God," I thought to myself, "How is it that none of the men have lost their hair but all the women are bald?"

I discovered chemo meds and treatments are different. The meds and treatment vary depending on the type of cancer you have. I will never forget my first treatment. What I experienced, and what I went through will stay with me forever.

The nurse began the treatment and walked away. My heart began to beat so fast that I went into a convulsion that caused an uncontrollable muscle spasm in my back. Thank God, for my daughter in Christ being there with me. She stopped the machine that administered the medicine in my veins and quickly went to get the nurse. I was calling on my doctor, Jesus. They discovered that I was allergic to the medicine. Every time after that I had a steroid and allergy medicine mix before starting my treatment. An alert was placed on my file to avoid this ever happening again.

Every time I was in the chemo chair, God showed me the hearts of the people in the room with me. God allowed me to feel in my spirit who was weak and who was strong. I would begin to pray for them and tried to have uplifting conversations with the ones that needed them. I prayed quietly with those who were withdrawn.

God is a healer of His people. I believe He can and will heal. All power belongs to God. Call on the name of Jesus. God said that He would never leave or forsake me. These were my thoughts when I began to pray for the strength to give in to the tricks and attacks of the enemy. Jesus encouraged me so I could in turn encourage others to talk with Him beyond the chemo chair. The Lord instructed and encouraged me to write down all my feelings and prayers in the midst of all that I was going through.

When you finish reading this book, I encourage you to pass it onto someone else that they might be encouraged. The number of cancer patients seems to be getting higher with each day. I want them to know that it is going to take prayer and praise to get them through the process. Remember, praise will bring you through. Praise Him!

"I reckon that the sufferings of this present time are not worthy to be compared with the glory, which shall be revealed in us." (Romans 8:18)

Days of Loneliness

I remember all the moments of loneliness. Sometimes you can be in a room full of people and still be lonely. Seems like no one understands that your days of shutdown are when you need a pick-me-up the most.

A pick-me-up could be a trip out of the house, a walk in the backyard, a phone call just to say, "I love you," a gift, a bouquet of flowers, Bible study in your quiet time, a girls day out, a makeover, or a movie with the family. When my family or friends would see me staring off in the distance, they would do things to make me feel like I had purpose. Love is the best medicine.

"Cast all your anxiety on Him,
because he cares for you." (1 Peter 5:7, NIV)

Words of Encouragement

When I gave all of my sickness to God, I would not allow doubt to enter into my spirit.

I would ask Him to make me a miracle and to never allow me to get sick while taking chemo. I did not see myself ever getting sick, so I never did. Everyone knows a person can only believe what he or she sees. 2 Corinthians 5:7 says, "We walk by faith, not by sight." If enough people keep telling you how you are supposed to feel, then at some point you will actually begin to feel that way.

The degree or measure of faith you possess will determine to what degree your level of strength will be. Trust and belief in God is what will help you to keep on living.

"For God so loved the world, that He gave His only begotten son, that whoever believes in Him should not perish but have everlasting life." (John 3:16)

It does not matter how bad the report from the doctor is trust God to deliver you. Believe that He *is* able.

Get with your prayer team after your doctor's appointment. Speak healing over your body and pray for one another.

"And they said, believe on the Lord Jesus Christ, and thou shalt be saved, and thy house," (Acts 16:31)

My Testimony

All I can say about my life, at this point in time, is PRAISE GOD! Somebody needs to bless the Lamb of God right now. God has been a friend and mother to me, a motherless woman. God has been the head doctor through it all. My battle with cancer would have never been won without Him.

From day one, the Lord was with me. He revealed to me that only He (God) could get me through this. Jesus has been my friend since childhood; since then I have felt His presence. When the doctor told me that I had cancer, I stepped out of the room to talk to Jesus. I said, *"God, I know you will get me through this."*

As I spoke with the Lord, I asked Him to make me His miracle patient. I asked the Lord to never let me be sick in the way of vomiting, diarrhea, and fever. He kept me! I never experienced any of what I had asked of God to spare me from. For that, I thank Him and am very grateful.

It seemed like a dream. My faith and trust in God had gotten stronger through my fight. I lost my hair. My body became weak. My fingernails fell off for seven days. I could not eat after chemo, sometimes for as many as seven days. I had to stay out of the sun. For ten days in a row, I had to give myself a shot in the stomach to treat blood clots. Through everything, I never stopped trusting in God's power. I knew that when I came out, I would be stronger than ever and healed by the blood of Jesus!

For three months of treatment, I was safe in the arms of Jesus. I had daily conversations with Him. I almost lost my church, but God made me a better pastor. My church and my ministry are not the same. They are greater. God gave me my own television show called *Churches United.* He put me on assignment to unite local churches. God has increased my territory by sending me to preach and fellowship with many churches. My life belongs to Him and I am so blessed to be alive. That is something I will never take for granted. I thank Him every day for my life, health, and strength.

"But as it is written, Eye hath not seen, nor ear heard, neither have entered into the heart of man, the things, which God hath prepared for them that love Him." (1 Corinthians 2:9)

Let Me Preach

(For Just A Minute)

We must give Him thanks.

Almighty God, give me a word of encouragement for your people. God I am willing to be used for Your glory. Thank you, God for my life, health, and strength. Amen!

Let us look at the people in the Bible who really needed Jesus, those who cried out to be healed or sought to be in His presence. Sometimes when our body is under attack, we will call the doctor for help. There is nothing wrong with this, but the doctor did not create you. Jesus did. This is why I always tell people to before the face of God.

God is our creator and designer. He is the author and finisher of all things. We must learn to take all things to Him first. Trust Him and know that He is able to do all things. Friends and loved ones will tell you that you are in a battle. But I am telling you to trust God and know in your heart that there is nothing too hard for God to do. This is not to say that God does not use doctors. But what I am saying is that you should take all things to God in prayer first.

"Be anxious for nothing, but in everything by prayer and supplication, with thanksgiving, let your request be made known to God and the peace of God which surpasses all understanding, will guard your hearts and mind through Christ Jesus." (Philippians 4:6-7)

Time to Get Your Life Back

Fear will kick in when cancer spreads. Every little cold or fever will put you in a place of worry, but you must glorify God in everything. Even in times of bad news, let your request be made known to God. The Father wants us to come to Him as children seeking love, help, and understanding from Him. You have got to believe in your spirit that all answers are in His hands.

Put your request before God. He is waiting to hear what your needs are. Believe that He can do anything. He will give you the peace you need to get through anything the body cannot handle. Philippians 4:6-7 reminds us that the peace of God surpasses all understanding. God already knows that we will have to go through certain things that we might not understand but His peace will guard our hearts and minds. Satan wants to trouble our mind with anxiety and depression. He wants to hurt the heart with sorrow, pain, and distress. All of these things will kill you faster than any cancer can.

When you read the Bible and get a clear understanding of God's love for us, your heart will draw closer to Him. God desires to hear your praise and worship of Him. How can we ask for things from Him and not be willing to give Him something in return for it? Sometimes God will give us a reason to remember why we should praise Him. Him carrying us through stages of illness and sickness is one of the ways He receives our praise.

We all are being tested in some way. There is an appointed time for all of us to die, but even death is in His hands. God is able to turn a situation that looks bad into something that can be used for His glory. Sometimes, God allows things to get bad in order for a miracle to take place. Your prayer life must be strong. Pray in the spirit with the Holy Spirit. Always talk to God. Testify to the angels as though you are looking right at them because they can see Jesus. As a matter of fact, let me stop and say a quick prayer for you right now. (I feel the presence of God right now):

Lord, I first want to say thank you! Thank you for allowing me to be of service to You, for Your glory. Help me, God, as I minister to Your people. I pray that this book and my testimony will encourage them to trust more in You. God, let your Holy Spirit sweep through their soul. Touch the sick right now with a warm feeling of love. Let every mind rest with peace. I ask these things in Jesus' name. Amen.

As you continue to fight, warring for your soul and good health, stay in the right atmosphere and stay positive. Remember, laughter is good for the bones and the soul. Watch a funny movie. Call someone who always brings a smile to your face. Never ask anyone to tell you how you look or whether *they* think you are going to make it through. Just trust in Jesus and pray for an answer to your prayers. I love you, and God loves you even more.

Just Keep Praising God

The Hebrew word for praise is *Yudah.* Praise is defined as an expression of admiration, to pay tribute to or to speak highly of someone or something. How do we praise God? By singing His praise, raving about His goodness, talking about His glory, dancing in the Holy Spirit, reading the book of Psalms, or simply giving thanks.

Never Give Up

Above all things, fight a good fight! I hope my prayers and testimony will help you to trust God even when the world says that there is no hope. Remember, even though I have not met you, I still love you! May God continue to bless and enrich your life!

All The Glory Belongs to God!

Where do I start? Lord God, Father of all creation, I love you. At first my life seemed so hard. Everything I have been through was for the glory of God. Even when I was sick as a child—always falling, getting cuts, and broken bones—You were always with me.

Thank you for teaching me how to pick myself up and grab hold of the strength that was leading to Your glory. There have been times when I wondered in my spirit, "Where would I be if I did not have the Lord on my side."

Thank you for showing me your glory an grace. I realize now, that *"all things work together for the good of those who love God, to those who are called according to his purpose."* (Romans 8:28). This is why I give you all the glory.

Thank you, God for bringing me, not only through cancer but also through life. We all must be tested and tried. When I lost my daughter, it was the saddest day of my life. Now, when I reflect back on the experience all I can see is the grace of God. For that, I give You praise. Psalm 30:5 says, *"Weeping may endure for a night but joy cometh in the morning."*

Great are Your works!

You are awesome and I cannot stop giving You praise. All that I am is because of You. Nothing is possible without You. I put all my trust in You because Your love for me and all people. You said, *"You will never leave me nor forsake me."* (Deuteronomy 31:6).

To God be the glory!

About The Author

Author Sandra G. Jones is a pastor, television host, and founder of *Churches United.* Based in Dublin, Georgia, Pastor Jones graduated from East Atlanta High School and the Atlanta Medical and Dental College.

She moved to Dublin, Georgia in 2003, where she received her call to the ministry. Her vision is to help unite the body of Christ through her many God-given gifts, to help awaken, encourage and impart knowledge to God's people.

Prayers beyond the

CHEMO CHAIR

Praise, Encouragement, & Testimony Journal

Praise

Praise

Praise

Praise

Praise

Praise

Praise

Praise

Praise

Praise

Praise

Praise

Praise

Praise

Praise

Encouragement

Encouragement

Encouragement ______________________

Encouragement

Encouragement

Encouragement

Encouragement

Encouragement

Encouragement ______________________

Encouragement

Encouragement

Encouragement

Encouragement

Encouragement ________________

Encouragement

Encouragement

Testimony

Testimony

Testimony

Testimony

Testimony

Testimony

Testimony

Testimony ________________________________

Testimony

Testimony

Testimony

Testimony

Testimony

Testimony

Testimony ______________________

www.ingramcontent.com/pod-product-compliance
Lightning Source LLC
Chambersburg PA
CBHW070448170726
48291CB00005B/1646
9781942871811